CW00455721

DASH DIET COOKBOOK

2021

The Guide to Lower your Blood Pressure for Healthy Living.

Quick and Easy Recipes with Delicious and Tasty Meals.

Low Sodium Dishes for Better Healthy Lifestyle.

Sandra Podolski

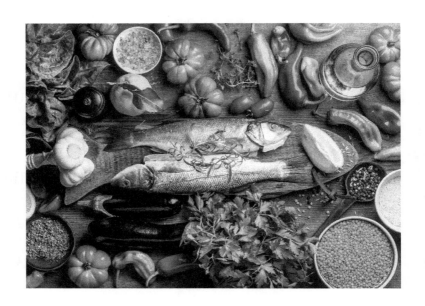

Table of Contents

Table of Contents	4
Chickpea Cauliflower Tikka Masala	11
Eggplant Parmesan Stacks	13
Roasted Vegetable Enchiladas	15
Lentil Avocado Tacos	18
Tomato & Olive Orecchiette with Basil Pesto	20
Italian Stuffed Portobello Mushroom Burgers	22
Gnocchi with Tomato Basil Sauce	24
Creamy Pumpkin Pasta	26
Mexican-Style Potato Casserole	28
Black Bean Stew with Cornbread	31
Mushroom Florentine	34
Hasselback Eggplant	36
Vegetarian Kebabs	37
White Beans Stew	39
Vegetarian Lasagna	41
Carrot Cakes	43
Vegan Chili	44
Aromatic Whole Grain Spaghetti	45
Chunky Tomatoes	46
Baked Falafel	48
Paella	50
Mushroom Cakes	52
Glazed Eggplant Rings	54
Sweet Potato Balls	56
Chickpea Curry	58
Pan-Fried Salmon with Salad	60
Veggie Variety	62

Vegetable Pasta 64

Vegetable Noodles with Bolognese 66

Harissa Bolognese with Vegetable Noodles 68

Curry Vegetable Noodles with Chicken 70

Sweet and Sour Vegetable Noodles 72

Tuna Sandwich 74

Fruited Quinoa Salad 76

Turkey Wrap 78

Chicken Wrap 79

Veggie Wrap 81

Salmon Wrap 83

Dill Chicken Salad 85

Side Dishes 87

Turmeric Endives 87

Parmesan Endives 89

Lemon Asparagus 91

Lime Carrots 93

Garlic Potato Pan 95

Balsamic Cabbage 97

Chili Broccoli 99

Hot Brussels Sprouts 101

Paprika Brussels Sprouts 103

Creamy Cauliflower Mash 105

Avocado, Tomato, and Olives Salad 107

The information in the following pages is broadly considered a truthful and accurate account of facts and as such, any inattention, use, or misuse of the information in question by the reader will render any resulting actions solely under their purview. There are no scenarios in which the publisher or the original author of this work can be in any fashion deemed liable for any hardship or damages that may befall them after undertaking information described herein.

Additionally, the information in the following pages is intended only for informational purposes and should thus be thought of as universal. As befitting its nature, it is presented without assurance regarding its prolonged validity or interim quality. Trademarks that are mentioned are done without written consent and can in no way be considered an endorsement from the trademark holder.

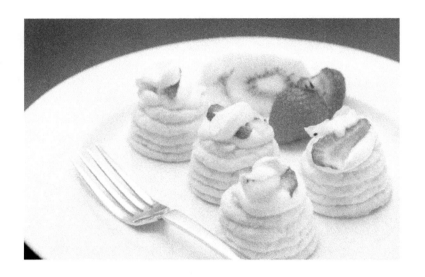

Chickpea Cauliflower Tikka Masala

Preparation time: 15 minutes

Cooking time: 40 minutes

Servings: 6

Ingredients:

- 2 tablespoons olive oil

- 1 yellow onion, peeled and diced

- 4 garlic cloves, peeled and minced

- 1-inch piece fresh ginger, peeled and minced

- 2 tablespoons Garam Masala

- 1 teaspoon kosher or sea salt

- ½ teaspoon ground black pepper

- ¼ teaspoon ground cayenne pepper

- ½ small head cauliflower, small florets

- 2 (15-ounce) cans no-salt-added chickpeas, rinsed and drained

- 1 (15-ounce) can no-salt-added petite diced tomatoes, drained

- 1½ cups unsalted vegetable broth

- ½ (15-ounce) can coconut milk

- Zest and juice of 1 lime

- ½ cup fresh cilantro leaves, chopped, divided

- 1½ cups cooked Fluffy Brown Rice, divided

Directions:

1. Warm-up olive oil over medium heat, then put the onion and sauté within 4 to 5 minutes in a large Dutch oven or stockpot. Stir in the garlic, ginger, garam masala, salt, black pepper, and cayenne pepper and toast for 30 to 60 seconds, until fragrant.

2. Stir in the cauliflower florets, chickpeas, diced tomatoes, and vegetable broth and increase to medium-high. Simmer within 15 minutes, until the cauliflower is fork-tender.

3. Remove, then stir in the coconut milk, lime juice, lime zest, and half of the cilantro. Taste and adjust the seasoning, if necessary. Serve over the rice and the remaining chopped cilantro.

Nutrition:

Calories: 323

Fat: 12g

Sodium: 444mg

Carbohydrate: 44g

Protein: 11g

Eggplant Parmesan Stacks

Preparation time: 15 minutes

Cooking time: 20 minutes

Servings: 4

Ingredients:

- 1 large eggplant, cut into thick slices

- 2 tablespoons olive oil, divided

- ¼ teaspoon kosher or sea salt

- ¼ teaspoon ground black pepper

- 1 cup panko bread crumbs

- ¼ cup freshly grated Parmesan cheese

- 5 to 6 garlic cloves, minced

- ½ pound fresh mozzarella, sliced

- 1½ cups lower-sodium marinara

- ½ cup fresh basil leaves, torn

Directions:

1. Preheat the oven to 425°F. Coat the eggplant slices in 1 tablespoon olive oil and sprinkle with the salt and black pepper. Put on a large baking sheet, then roast for 10 to 12 minutes, until soft with crispy

edges. Remove the eggplant and set the oven to a low broil.

2. In a bowl, stir the remaining tablespoon of olive oil, bread crumbs, Parmesan cheese, and garlic. Remove the cooled eggplant from the baking sheet and clean it.

3. Create layers on the same baking sheet by stacking a roasted eggplant slice with a slice of mozzarella, a tablespoon of marinara, and a tablespoon of the bread crumb mixture, repeating with 2 layers of each ingredient. Cook under the broiler within 3 to 4 minutes until the cheese is melted and bubbly.

Nutrition:

Calories: 377

Fat: 22g

Sodium: 509mg

Carbohydrate: 29g

Protein: 16g

Roasted Vegetable Enchiladas

Preparation time: 15 minutes

Cooking time: 45 minutes

Servings: 8

Ingredients:

- 2 zucchinis, diced

- 1 red bell pepper, seeded and sliced

- 1 red onion, peeled and sliced

- 2 ears corn

- 2 tablespoons canola oil

- 1 can no-salt-added black beans, drained

- 1½ tablespoons chili powder

- 2 teaspoon ground cumin

- 1/8 teaspoon kosher or sea salt

- ½ teaspoon ground black pepper

- 8 (8-inch) whole-wheat tortillas

- 1 cup Enchilada Sauce or store-bought enchilada sauce

- ½ cup shredded Mexican-style cheese

- ½ cup plain nonfat Greek yogurt

- ½ cup cilantro leaves, chopped

Directions:

1. Preheat oven to 400°F. Place the zucchini, red bell pepper, and red onion on a baking sheet. Place the ears of corn separately on the same baking sheet. Drizzle all with the canola oil and toss to coat. Roast for 10 to 12 minutes, until the vegetables are tender. Remove and reduce the temperature to 375°F.

2. Cut the corn from the cob. Transfer the corn kernels, zucchini, red bell pepper, and onion to a bowl and stir in the black beans, chili powder, cumin, salt, and black pepper until combined.

3. Oiled a 9-by-13-inch baking dish with cooking spray. Line up the tortillas in the greased baking dish. Evenly distribute the vegetable bean filling into each tortilla. Pour half of the enchilada sauce and sprinkle half of the shredded cheese on top of the filling.

4. Roll each tortilla into enchilada shape and place them seam-side down. Pour the remaining enchilada sauce and sprinkle the remaining cheese over the enchiladas. Bake for 25 minutes until the cheese is melted and bubbly. Serve the enchiladas with Greek yogurt and chopped cilantro.

Nutrition:

Calories: 335

Fat: 15g

Sodium: 557mg

Carbohydrate: 42g

Protein: 13g

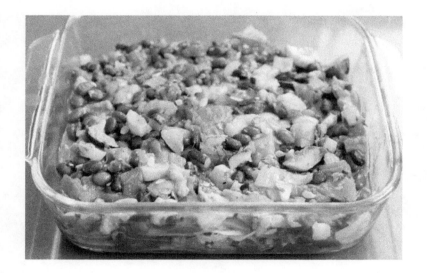

Lentil Avocado Tacos

Preparation time: 15 minutes

Cooking time: 35 minutes

Servings: 6

Ingredients:

- 1 tablespoon canola oil

- ½ yellow onion, peeled and diced

- 2-3 garlic cloves, minced

- 1½ cups dried lentils

- ½ teaspoon kosher or sea salt

- 3 to 3½ cups unsalted vegetable or chicken stock

- 2½ tablespoons Taco Seasoning or store-bought low-sodium taco seasoning

- 16 (6-inch) corn tortillas, toasted

- 2 ripe avocados, peeled and sliced

Directions:

1. Heat-up the canola oil in a large skillet or Dutch oven over medium heat. Cook the onion within 4 to 5 minutes, until soft. Mix in the garlic and cook within 30 seconds until fragrant. Then add the

lentils, salt, and stock. Bring to a simmer for 25 to 35 minutes, adding additional stock if needed.

2. When there's only a small amount of liquid left in the pan, and the lentils are al dente, stir in the taco seasoning and let simmer for 1 to 2 minutes. Taste and adjust the seasoning, if necessary. Spoon the lentil mixture into tortillas and serve with the avocado slices.

Nutrition:

Calories: 400

Fat: 14g

Sodium: 336mg

Carbohydrate: 64g

Fiber: 15g

Protein: 16g

Tomato & Olive Orecchiette with Basil Pesto

Preparation time: 15 minutes

Cooking time: 25 minutes

Servings: 6

Ingredients:

- 12 ounces orecchiette pasta

- 2 tablespoons olive oil

- 1-pint cherry tomatoes, quartered

- ½ cup Basil Pesto or store-bought pesto

- ¼ cup kalamata olives, sliced

- 1 tablespoon dried oregano leaves

- ¼ teaspoon kosher or sea salt

- ½ teaspoon freshly cracked black pepper

- ¼ teaspoon crushed red pepper flakes

- 2 tablespoons freshly grated Parmesan cheese

Directions:

1. Boil a large pot of water. Cook the orecchiette, drain and transfer the pasta to a large nonstick skillet.

2. Put the skillet over medium-low heat, then heat the olive oil. Stir in the cherry tomatoes, pesto, olives, oregano, salt, black pepper, and crushed red pepper flakes. Cook within 8 to 10 minutes, until heated throughout. Serve the pasta with the freshly grated Parmesan cheese.

Nutrition:

Calories: 332

Fat: 13g

Sodium: 389mg

Carbohydrate: 44g

Protein: 9g

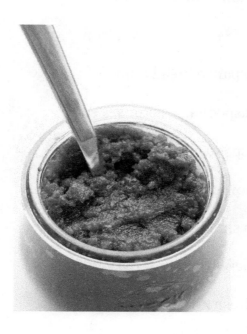

Italian Stuffed Portobello Mushroom Burgers

Preparation time: 15 minutes

Cooking time: 25 minutes

Servings: 4

Ingredients:

- 1 tablespoon olive oil

- 4 large portobello mushrooms, washed and dried

- ½ yellow onion, peeled and diced

- 4 garlic cloves, peeled and minced

- 1 can cannellini beans, drained

- ½ cup fresh basil leaves, torn

- ½ cup panko bread crumbs

- 1/8 teaspoon kosher or sea salt

- ¼ teaspoon ground black pepper

- 1 cup lower-sodium marinara, divided

- ½ cup shredded mozzarella cheese

- 4 whole-wheat buns, toasted

- 1 cup fresh arugula

Directions:

1. Heat-up the olive oil in a large skillet to medium-high heat. Sear the mushrooms for 4 to 5 minutes per side, until slightly soft. Place on a baking sheet. Preheat the oven to a low broil.

2. Put the onion in the skillet and cook for 4 to 5 minutes, until slightly soft. Mix in the garlic then cooks within 30 to 60 seconds. Move the onions plus garlic to a bowl. Add the cannellini beans and smash with the back of a fork to form a chunky paste. Stir in the basil, bread crumbs, salt, and black pepper and half of the marinara. Cook for 5 minutes.

3. Remove the bean mixture from the stove and divide among the mushroom caps. Spoon the remaining marinara over the stuffed mushrooms and top each with the mozzarella cheese. Broil within 3 to 4 minutes, until the cheese is melted and bubbly. Transfer the burgers to the toasted whole-wheat buns and top with the arugula.

Nutrition:

Calories: 407

Fat: 9g

Sodium: 575mg

Carbohydrate: 63g

Protein: 25g

Gnocchi with Tomato Basil Sauce

Preparation time: 15 minutes

Cooking time: 25 minutes

Servings: 6

Ingredients:

- 2 tablespoons olive oil

- ½ yellow onion, peeled and diced

- 3 cloves garlic, peeled and minced

- 1 (32-ounce) can no-salt-added crushed San Marzano tomatoes

- ¼ cup fresh basil leaves

- 2 teaspoons Italian seasoning

- ½ teaspoon kosher or sea salt

- 1 teaspoon granulated sugar

- ½ teaspoon ground black pepper

- 1/8 teaspoon crushed red pepper flakes

- 1 tablespoon heavy cream (optional)

- 12 ounces gnocchi

- ¼ cup freshly grated Parmesan cheese

Directions:

1. Heat-up the olive oil in a Dutch oven or stockpot over medium heat. Add the onion and sauté for 5 to 6 minutes, until soft. Stir in the garlic and stir until fragrant, 30 to 60 seconds. Then stir in the tomatoes, basil, Italian seasoning, salt, sugar, black pepper, and crushed red pepper flakes.

2. Bring to a simmer for 15 minutes. Stir in the heavy cream, if desired. For a smooth, puréed sauce, use an immersion blender or transfer sauce to a blender and purée until smooth. Taste and adjust the seasoning, if necessary.

3. While the sauce simmers, cook the gnocchi according to the package instructions, remove with a slotted spoon, and transfer to 6 bowls. Pour the sauce over the gnocchi and top with the Parmesan cheese.

Nutrition:

Calories: 287

Fat: 7g

Sodium: 527mg

Carbohydrate: 41g

Protein: 10g

Creamy Pumpkin Pasta

Preparation time: 15 minutes

Cooking time: 30 minutes

Servings: 6

Ingredients:

- 1-pound whole-grain linguine

- 1 tablespoon olive oil

- 3 garlic cloves, peeled and minced

- 2 tablespoons chopped fresh sage

- 1½ cups pumpkin purée

- 1 cup unsalted vegetable stock

- ½ cup low-fat evaporated milk

- ¾ teaspoon kosher or sea salt

- ½ teaspoon ground black pepper

- ½ teaspoon ground nutmeg

- ¼ teaspoon ground cayenne pepper

- ½ cup freshly grated Parmesan cheese, divided

Directions:

1. Cook the whole-grain linguine in a large pot of boiled water. Reserve ½ cup of pasta water and drain the rest. Set the pasta aside.

2. Warm-up olive oil over medium heat in a large skillet. Add the garlic and sage and sauté for 1 to 2 minutes, until soft and fragrant. Whisk in the pumpkin purée, stock, milk, and reserved pasta water and simmer for 4 to 5 minutes, until thickened.

3. Whisk in the salt, black pepper, nutmeg, and cayenne pepper and half of the Parmesan cheese. Stir in the cooked whole-grain linguine. Evenly divide the pasta among 6 bowls and top with the remaining Parmesan cheese.

Nutrition:
Calories: 381
Fat: 8g
Sodium: 175mg
Carbohydrate: 63g
Protein: 15g

Mexican-Style Potato Casserole

Preparation time: 15 minutes

Cooking time: 60 minutes

Servings: 8

Ingredients:

- Cooking spray

- 2 tablespoons canola oil

- ½ yellow onion, peeled and diced

- 4 garlic cloves, peeled and minced

- 2 tablespoons all-purpose flour

- 1¼ cups milk

- 1 tablespoon chili powder

- ½ tablespoon ground cumin

- 1 teaspoon kosher salt or sea salt

- ½ teaspoon ground black pepper

- ¼ teaspoon ground cayenne pepper

- 1½ cups shredded Mexican-style cheese, divided

- 1 (4-ounce) can green chilis, drained

- 1½ pounds baby Yukon Gold or red potatoes, thinly sliced

- 1 red bell pepper, thinly sliced

Directions:

1. Preheat the oven to 400°F. Oiled a 9-by-13-inch baking dish with cooking spray. In a large saucepan, warm canola oil on medium heat. Add the onion and sauté for 4 to 5 minutes, until soft. Mix in the garlic, then cook until fragrant, 30 to 60 seconds.

2. Mix in the flour, then put in the milk while whisking. Slow simmer for about 5 minutes, until thickened. Whisk in the chili powder, cumin, salt, black pepper, and cayenne pepper.

3. Remove from the heat and whisk in half of the shredded cheese and the green chilis. Taste and adjust the seasoning, if necessary. Line up one-third of the sliced potatoes and sliced bell pepper in the baking dish and top with a quarter of the remaining shredded cheese.

4. Repeat with 2 more layers. Pour the cheese sauce over the top and sprinkle with the remaining shredded cheese. Cover it with aluminum foil and bake within 45 to 50 minutes, until the potatoes are tender.

5. Remove the foil and bake again within 5 to 10 minutes, until the topping is slightly browned. Let

cool within 20 minutes before slicing into 8 pieces. Serve.

Nutrition:

Calories: 195

Fat: 10g

Sodium: 487mg

Carbohydrate: 19g

Protein: 8g

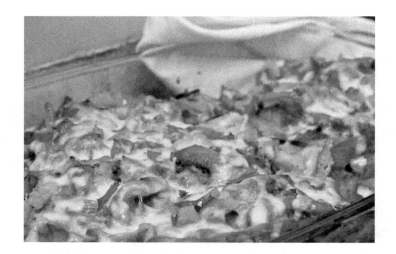

Black Bean Stew with Cornbread

Preparation time: 15 minutes

Cooking time: 55 minutes

Servings: 6

Ingredients:

For the black bean stew:

- 2 tablespoons canola oil

- 1 yellow onion, peeled and diced

- 4 garlic cloves, peeled and minced

- 1 tablespoon chili powder

- 1 tablespoon ground cumin

- ¼ teaspoon kosher or sea salt

- ½ teaspoon ground black pepper

- 2 cans no-salt-added black beans, drained

- 1 (10-ounce) can fire-roasted diced tomatoes

- ½ cup fresh cilantro leaves, chopped

For the cornbread topping:

- 1¼ cups cornmeal

- ½ cup all-purpose flour

- ½ teaspoon baking powder

- ¼ teaspoon baking soda

- 1/8 teaspoon kosher or sea salt

- 1 cup low-fat buttermilk

- 2 tablespoons honey

- 1 large egg

Directions:

1. Warm-up canola oil over medium heat in a large Dutch oven or stockpot. Add the onion and sauté for 4 to 6 minutes, until the onion is soft. Stir in the garlic, chili powder, cumin, salt, and black pepper.

2. Cook within 1 to 2 minutes, until fragrant. Add the black beans and diced tomatoes. Bring to a simmer and cook for 15 minutes. Remove, then stir in the fresh cilantro. Taste and adjust the seasoning, if necessary.

3. Preheat the oven to 375°F. While the stew simmers, prepare the cornbread topping. Mix the cornmeal, baking soda, flour, baking powder, plus salt in a bowl. In a measuring cup, whisk the buttermilk, honey, and egg until combined. Put the batter into the dry fixing until just combined.

4. In oven-safe bowls or dishes, spoon out the black bean soup. Distribute dollops of the cornbread

batter on top and then spread it out evenly with a spatula. Bake within 30 minutes, until the cornbread is just set.

Nutrition:

Calories: 359

Fat: 7g

Sodium: 409mg

Carbohydrate: 61g

Protein: 14g

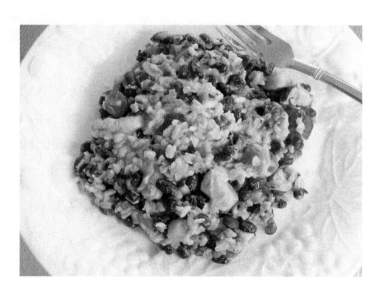

Mushroom Florentine

Preparation time: 15 minutes

Cooking time: 20 minutes

Servings: 4

Ingredients:

- 5 oz whole-grain pasta

- ¼ cup low-sodium vegetable broth

- 1 cup mushrooms, sliced

- ¼ cup of soy milk

- 1 teaspoon olive oil

- ½ teaspoon Italian seasonings

Directions:

1. Cook the pasta according to the direction of the manufacturer. Then pour olive oil into the saucepan and heat it. Add mushrooms and Italian seasonings. Stir the mushrooms well and cook for 10 minutes.

2. Then add soy milk and vegetable broth. Add cooked pasta and mix up the mixture well. Cook it for 5 minutes on low heat.

Nutrition:

Calories 287

Protein 12.4g

Carbohydrates 50.4g

Fat 4.2g

Sodium 26mg

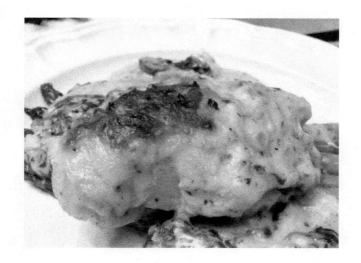

Hasselback Eggplant

Preparation time: 15 minutes

Cooking time: 25 minutes

Servings: 2

Ingredients:

- 2 eggplants, trimmed

- 2 tomatoes, sliced

- 1 tablespoon low-fat yogurt

- 1 teaspoon curry powder

- 1 teaspoon olive oil

Directions:

1. Make the cuts in the eggplants in the shape of the Hasselback. Then rub the vegetables with curry powder and fill with sliced tomatoes. Sprinkle the eggplants with olive oil and yogurt and wrap in the foil (each Hasselback eggplant wrap separately). Bake the vegetables at 375F for 25 minutes.

Nutrition:

Calories 188

Protein 7g

Carbohydrates 38.1g

Fat 3g

Sodium 23mg

Vegetarian Kebabs

Preparation time: 15 minutes

Cooking time: 6 minutes

Servings: 4

Ingredients:

- 2 tablespoons balsamic vinegar

- 1 tablespoon olive oil

- 1 teaspoon dried parsley

- 2 tablespoons water

- 2 sweet peppers

- 2 red onions, peeled

- 2 zucchinis, trimmed

Directions:

1. Cut the sweet peppers and onions into medium size squares. Then slice the zucchini. String all vegetables into the skewers. After this, in the shallow bowl, mix up olive oil, dried parsley, water, and balsamic vinegar.

2. Sprinkle the vegetable skewers with olive oil mixture and transfer in the preheated to 390F grill. Cook the kebabs within 3 minutes per side or until the vegetables are light brown.

Nutrition:

Calories 88

Protein 2.4g

Carbohydrates 13g

Fat 3.9g

Sodium 14mg

White Beans Stew

Preparation time: 15 minutes
Cooking time: 55 minutes
Servings: 4
Ingredients:

- 1 cup white beans, soaked

- 1 cup low-sodium vegetable broth

- 1 cup zucchini, chopped

- 1 teaspoon tomato paste

- 1 tablespoon avocado oil

- 4 cups of water

- ½ teaspoon peppercorns

- ½ teaspoon ground black pepper

- ¼ teaspoon ground nutmeg

Directions:

1. Heat avocado oil in the saucepan, add zucchinis, and roast them for 5 minutes. After this, add white beans, vegetable broth, tomato paste, water, peppercorns, ground black pepper, and ground nutmeg. Simmer the stew within 50 minutes on low heat.

Nutrition:

Calories 184

Protein 12.3g

Carbohydrates 32.6g

Fat 1g

Sodium 55mg

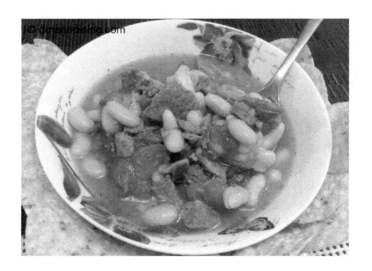

Vegetarian Lasagna

Preparation time: 15 minutes

Cooking time: 30 minutes

Servings: 6

Ingredients:

- 1 cup carrot, diced

- ½ cup bell pepper, diced

- 1 cup spinach, chopped

- 1 tablespoon olive oil

- 1 teaspoon chili powder

- 1 cup tomatoes, chopped

- 4 oz low-fat cottage cheese

- 1 eggplant, sliced

- 1 cup low-sodium vegetable broth

Directions:

1. Put carrot, bell pepper, and spinach in the saucepan. Add olive oil and chili powder and stir the vegetables well. Cook them for 5 minutes.

2. Make the sliced eggplant layer in the casserole mold and top it with vegetable mixture. Add tomatoes,

vegetable stock, and cottage cheese. Bake the lasagna for 30 minutes at 375F.

Nutrition:

Calories 77

Protein 4.1g

Carbohydrates 9.7g

Fat 3g

Sodium 124mg

Carrot Cakes

Preparation time: 15 minutes

Cooking time: 10 minutes

Servings: 4

Ingredients:

- 1 cup carrot, grated

- 1 tablespoon semolina

- 1 egg, beaten

- 1 teaspoon Italian seasonings

- 1 tablespoon sesame oil

Directions:

1. In the mixing bowl, mix up grated carrot, semolina, egg, and Italian seasonings. Heat sesame oil in the skillet. Make the carrot cakes with the help of 2 spoons and put in the skillet. Roast the cakes for 4 minutes per side.

Nutrition:

Calories 70

Protein 1.9g

Carbohydrates 4.8g

Fat 4.9g

Sodium 35mg

Vegan Chili

Preparation time: 15 minutes

Cooking time: 25 minutes

Servings: 4

Ingredients:

- ½ cup bulgur

- 1 cup tomatoes, chopped

- 1 chili pepper, chopped

- 1 cup red kidney beans, cooked

- 2 cups low-sodium vegetable broth

- 1 teaspoon tomato paste

- ½ cup celery stalk, chopped

Directions:

1. Put all ingredients in the big saucepan and stir well. Close the lid and simmer the chili for 25 minutes over medium-low heat.

Nutrition:

Calories 234

Protein 13.1g

Carbohydrates 44.9g

Fat 0.9g

Sodium 92mg

Aromatic Whole Grain Spaghetti

Preparation time: 15 minutes

Cooking time: 10 minutes

Servings: 2

Ingredients:

- 1 teaspoon dried basil

- ¼ cup of soy milk

- 6 oz whole-grain spaghetti

- 2 cups of water

- 1 teaspoon ground nutmeg

Directions:

1. Bring the water to boil, add spaghetti, and cook them for 8-10 minutes. Meanwhile, bring the soy milk to boil. Drain the cooked spaghetti and mix them up with soy milk, ground nutmeg, and dried basil. Stir the meal well.

Nutrition:

Calories 128

Protein 5.6g

Carbohydrates 25g

Fat 1.4g

Sodium 25mg

Chunky Tomatoes

Preparation time: 15 minutes

Cooking time: 15 minutes

Servings: 3

Ingredients:

- 2 cups plum tomatoes, roughly chopped

- ½ cup onion, diced

- ½ teaspoon garlic, diced

- 1 teaspoon Italian seasonings

- 1 teaspoon canola oil

- 1 chili pepper, chopped

Directions:

1. Heat canola oil in the saucepan. Add chili pepper and onion. Cook the vegetables for 5 minutes. Stir them from time to time. After this, add tomatoes, garlic, and Italian seasonings. Close the lid and sauté the dish for 10 minutes.

Nutrition:

Calories 550

Protein 1.7g

Carbohydrates 8.4g

Fat 2.3g

Sodium 17mg

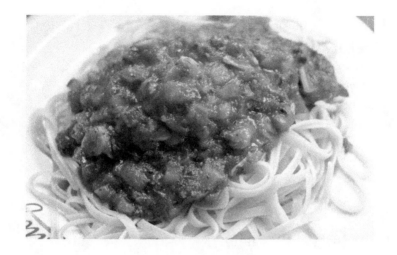

Baked Falafel

Preparation time: 15 minutes

Cooking time: 25 minutes

Servings: 6

Ingredients:

- 2 cups chickpeas, cooked

- 1 yellow onion, diced

- 3 tablespoons olive oil

- 1 cup fresh parsley, chopped

- 1 teaspoon ground cumin

- ½ teaspoon coriander

- 2 garlic cloves, diced

Directions:

1. Blend all fixing in the food processor. Preheat the oven to 375F. Then line the baking tray with the baking paper. Make the balls from the chickpeas mixture and press them gently in the shape of the falafel. Put the falafel in the tray and bake in the oven for 25 minutes.

Nutrition:

Calories 316

Protein 13.5g

Carbohydrates 43.3g

Fat 11.2g

Fiber 12.4g

Sodium 23mg

Paella

Preparation time: 15 minutes

Cooking time: 25 minutes

Servings: 6

Ingredients:

- 1 teaspoon dried saffron

- 1 cup short-grain rice

- 1 tablespoon olive oil

- 2 cups of water

- 1 teaspoon chili flakes

- 6 oz artichoke hearts, chopped

- ½ cup green peas

- 1 onion, sliced

- 1 cup bell pepper, sliced

Directions:

1. Pour water into the saucepan. Add rice and cook it for 15 minutes. Meanwhile, heat olive oil in the skillet. Add dried saffron, chili flakes, onion, and bell pepper. Roast the vegetables for 5 minutes.

2. Add them to the cooked rice. Then add artichoke hearts and green peas. Stir the paella well and cook it for 10 minutes over low heat.

Nutrition:

Calories 170

Protein 4.2g

Carbohydrates 32.7g

Fat 2.7g

Sodium 33mg

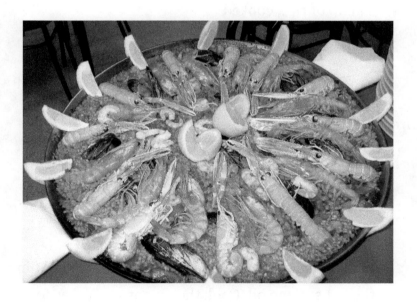

Mushroom Cakes

Preparation time: 15 minutes

Cooking time: 10 minutes

Servings: 4

Ingredients:

- 2 cups mushrooms, chopped

- 3 garlic cloves, chopped

- 1 tablespoon dried dill

- 1 egg, beaten

- ¼ cup of rice, cooked

- 1 tablespoon sesame oil

- 1 teaspoon chili powder

Directions:

1. Grind the mushrooms in the food processor. Add garlic, dill, egg, rice, and chili powder. Blend the mixture for 10 seconds. After this, heat sesame oil for 1 minute.

2. Make the medium size mushroom cakes and put in the hot sesame oil. Cook the mushroom cakes for 5 minutes per side on medium heat.

Nutrition:

Calories 103

Protein 3.7g

Carbohydrates 12g

Fat 4.8g

Sodium 27mg

Glazed Eggplant Rings

Preparation time: 15 minutes

Cooking time: 10 minutes

Servings: 4

Ingredients:

- 3 eggplants, sliced

- 1 tablespoon liquid honey

- 1 teaspoon minced ginger

- 2 tablespoons lemon juice

- 3 tablespoons avocado oil

- ½ teaspoon ground coriander

- 3 tablespoons water

Directions:

1. Rub the eggplants with ground coriander. Then heat the avocado oil in the skillet for 1 minute. When the oil is hot, add the sliced eggplant and arrange it in one layer.

2. Cook the vegetables for 1 minute per side. Transfer the eggplant to the bowl. Then add minced ginger, liquid honey, lemon juice, and water in the skillet. Bring it to boil and add cooked eggplants. Coat the

vegetables in the sweet liquid well and cook for 2 minutes more.

Nutrition:

Calories 136

Protein 4.3g

Carbohydrates 29.6g

Fat 2.2g

Sodium 11mg

Sweet Potato Balls

Preparation time: 15 minutes

Cooking time: 10 minutes

Servings: 4

Ingredients:

- 1 cup sweet potato, mashed, cooked

- 1 tablespoon fresh cilantro, chopped

- 1 egg, beaten

- 3 tablespoons ground oatmeal

- 1 teaspoon ground paprika

- ½ teaspoon ground turmeric

- 2 tablespoons coconut oil

Directions:

1. Mix mashed sweet potato, fresh cilantro, egg, ground oatmeal, paprika, and turmeric in a bowl. Stir the mixture until smooth and make the small balls. Heat the coconut oil in the saucepan. Put the sweet potato balls, then cook them until golden brown.

Nutrition:

Calories 133

Protein 2.8g

Carbohydrates 13.1g

Fat 8.2g

Sodium 44mg

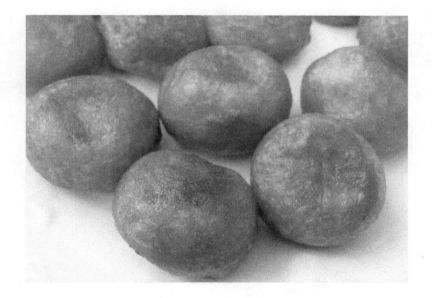

Chickpea Curry

Preparation time: 15 minutes

Cooking time: 10 minutes

Servings: 4

Ingredients:

- 1 ½ cup chickpeas, boiled

- 1 teaspoon curry powder

- ½ teaspoon garam masala

- 1 cup spinach, chopped

- 1 teaspoon coconut oil

- ¼ cup of soy milk

- 1 tablespoon tomato paste

- ½ cup of water

Directions:

1. Heat coconut oil in the saucepan. Add curry powder, garam masala, tomato paste, and soy milk. Whisk the mixture until smooth and bring it to boil.

2. Add water, spinach, and chickpeas. Stir the meal and close the lid. Cook it within 5 minutes over medium heat.

Nutrition:

Calories 298

Protein 15.4g

Carbohydrates 47.8g

Fat 6.1g

Sodium 37mg

Pan-Fried Salmon with Salad

Preparation time: 15 minutes

Cooking time: 20 minutes

Servings: 4

Ingredients:

- Pinch of salt and pepper

- 1 tablespoon extra-virgin olive oil

- 2 tablespoon unsalted butter

- ½ teaspoon fresh dill

- 1 tablespoon fresh lemon juice

- 100g salad leaves, or bag of mixed leaves

- Salad Dressing:

- 3 tablespoons olive oil

- 2 tablespoons balsamic vinaigrette

- 1/2 teaspoon maple syrup (honey)

Directions:

1. Pat-dry the salmon fillets with a paper towel and season with a pinch of salt and pepper. In a skillet, warm-up oil over medium-high heat and add fillets. Cook each side within 5 to 7 minutes until golden brown.

2. Dissolve butter, dill, and lemon juice in a small saucepan. Put the butter mixture onto the cooked salmon. Lastly, combine all the salad dressing ingredients and drizzle to mixed salad leaves in a large bowl. Toss to coat. Serve with fresh salads on the side. Enjoy!

Nutrition:

Calories 307

Fat 22g

Protein 34.6g

Sodium 80mg

Carbohydrate 1.7g

Veggie Variety

Preparation time: 15 minutes

Cooking time: 15 minutes

Servings: 2

Ingredients:

- ½ onion, diced

- 1 teaspoon vegetable oil (corn or sunflower oil)

- 200 g Tofu/ bean curd

- 4 cherry tomatoes, halved

- 30ml vegetable milk (soy or oat milk)

- ½ tsp curry powder

- 0.25 tsp paprika

- Pinch of Salt & Pepper

- 2 slices of Vegan protein bread/ Whole grain bread

- Chives for garnish

Directions:

1. Dice the onion and fry in a frying pan with the oil. Break the tofu by hand into small pieces and put them in the pan. Sauté 7-8 min. Season with curry, paprika, salt, and pepper. The cherry tomatoes and milk and cook it all over roast a few minutes. Serve

with bread as desired and sprinkle with chopped chives.

Nutrition:
Calories 216
Fat 8.4g
Protein 14.1g
Sodium 140mg
Carbohydrate 24.8g

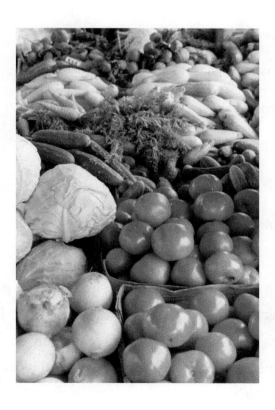

Vegetable Pasta

Preparation time: 15 minutes

Cooking time: 15 minutes

Servings: 4

Ingredients:

- 1 kg of thin zucchini

- 20 g of fresh ginger

- 350g smoked tofu

- 1 lime

- 2 cloves of garlic

- 2 tbsp sunflower oil

- 2 tablespoons of sesame seeds

- Pinch of salt and pepper

- 4 tablespoons fried onions

Directions:

1. Wash and clean the zucchini and, using a julienne cutter, cut the pulp around the kernel into long thin strips (noodles). Ginger peel and finely chop. Crumble tofu. Halve lime, squeeze juice. Peel and chop garlic.

2. Warm-up 1 tbsp of oil in a large pan and fry the tofu for about 5 minutes. After about 3 minutes, add ginger, garlic, and sesame. Season with soy sauce. Remove from the pan and keep warm.

3. Wipe out the pan, then warm 2 tablespoons of oil in it. Stir fry zucchini strips for about 4 minutes while turning. Season with salt, pepper, and lime juice. Arrange pasta and tofu. Sprinkle with fried onions.

Nutrition:

Calories 262

Fat 17.7g

Protein 15.4g

Sodium 62mg

Carbohydrate 17.1g

Vegetable Noodles with Bolognese

Preparation time: 15 minutes

Cooking time: 15 minutes

Servings: 4

Ingredients:

- 1.5 kg of small zucchini (e.g., green and yellow)

- 600g of carrots

- 1 onion

- 1 tbsp olive oil

- 250g of beef steak

- Pinch of Salt and pepper

- 2 tablespoons tomato paste

- 1 tbsp flour

- 1 teaspoon vegetable broth (instant)

- 40g pecorino or parmesan

- 1 small potty of basil

Directions:

1. Clean and peel zucchini and carrots and wash. Using a sharp, long knife, cut first into thin slices, then into long, fine strips. Clean or peel the soup greens, wash and cut into tiny cubes. Peel the onion and

chop finely. Heat the Bolognese oil in a large pan. Fry hack in it crumbly. Season with salt and pepper.

2. Briefly sauté the prepared vegetable and onion cubes. Stir in tomato paste. Dust the flour, sweat briefly. Pour in 400 ml of water and stir in the vegetable stock. Boil everything, simmer for 7-8 minutes.

3. Meanwhile, cook the vegetable strips in plenty of salted water for 3-5 minutes. Drain, collecting some cooking water. Add the vegetable strips to the pan and mix well. If the sauce is not liquid enough, stir in some vegetable cooking water and season everything again.

4. Slicing cheese into fine shavings. Wash the basil, shake dry, peel off the leaves, and cut roughly. Arrange vegetable noodles, sprinkle with parmesan and basil

Nutrition:

Calories 269

Fat 9.7g

Protein 25.6g

Sodium 253mg

Carbohydrate 21.7g

Harissa Bolognese with Vegetable Noodles

Preparation time: 15 minutes

Cooking time: 30 minutes

Servings: 4

Ingredients:

- 2 onions

- 1 clove of garlic

- 3-4 tbsp oil

- 400g ground beef

- Pinch salt, pepper, cinnamon

- 1 tsp Harissa (Arabic seasoning paste, tube)

- 1 tablespoon tomato paste

- 2 sweet potatoes

- 2 medium Zucchini

- 3 stems/basil

- 100g of feta

Directions:

1. Peel onions and garlic, finely dice. Warm-up 1 tbsp of oil in a wide saucepan. Fry hack in it crumbly. Fry

onions and garlic for a short time. Season with salt, pepper, and ½ teaspoon cinnamon. Stir in harissa and tomato paste.

2. Add tomatoes and 200 ml of water, bring to the boil and simmer for about 15 minutes with occasional stirring. Peel sweet potatoes and zucchini or clean and wash. Cut vegetables into spaghetti with a spiral cutter.

3. Warm-up 2-3 tablespoons of oil in a large pan. Braise sweet potato spaghetti in it for about 3 minutes. Add the zucchini spaghetti and continue to simmer for 3-4 minutes while turning.

4. Season with salt and pepper. Wash the basil, shake dry and peel off the leaves. Garnish vegetable spaghetti and Bolognese on plates. Feta crumbles over. Sprinkle with basil.

Nutrition:
Calories 452
Fat 22.3g
Protein 37.1g
Sodium 253mg
Carbohydrate 27.6g

Curry Vegetable Noodles with Chicken

Preparation time: 15 minutes

Cooking time: 15 minutes

Servings: 2

Ingredients:

- 600g of zucchini

- 500g chicken fillet

- Pinch of salt and pepper

- 2 tbsp oil

- 150 g of red and yellow cherry tomatoes

- 1 teaspoon curry powder

- 150g fat-free cheese

- 200 ml vegetable broth

- 4 stalk (s) of fresh basil

Directions:

1. Wash the zucchini, clean, and cut into long thin strips with a spiral cutter. Wash meat, pat dry, and season with salt. Heat 1 tbsp oil in a pan. Roast chicken in it for about 10 minutes until golden brown.

2. Wash cherry tomatoes and cut in half. Approximately 3 minutes before the end of the cooking time to the chicken in the pan. Heat 1 tbsp oil in another pan. Sweat curry powder into it then stirs in cream cheese and broth. Flavor the sauce with salt plus pepper and simmer for about 4 minutes.

3. Wash the basil, shake it dry and pluck the leaves from the stems. Cut small leaves of 3 stems. Remove meat from the pan and cut it into strips. Add tomatoes, basil, and zucchini to the sauce and heat for 2-3 minutes. Serve vegetable noodles and meat on plates and garnish with basil.

Nutrition:

Calories 376

Fat 17.2g

Protein 44.9g

Sodium 352mg

Carbohydrate 9.5

Cholesterol 53mg

Sweet and Sour Vegetable Noodles

Preparation time: 15 minutes

Cooking time: 30 minutes

Servings: 4

Ingredients:

- 4 chicken fillets (75 g each)

- 300g of whole-wheat spaghetti

- 750g carrots

- ½ liter clear chicken broth (instant)

- 1 tablespoon sugar

- 1 tbsp of green peppercorns

- 2-3 tbsp balsamic vinegar

- Capuchin flowers

- Pinch of salt

Directions:

1. Cook spaghetti in boiling water for about 8 minutes. Then drain. In the meantime, peel and wash carrots. Cut into long strips (best with a special grater). Blanch within 2 minutes in boiling salted water, drain. Wash chicken fillets. Add to the boiling chicken soup and cook for about 15 minutes.

2. Melt the sugar until golden brown. Measure 1/4 liter of chicken stock and deglaze the sugar with it. Add peppercorns, cook for 2 minutes. Season with salt and vinegar. Add the fillets, then cut into thin slices. Then turn the pasta and carrots in the sauce and serve garnished with capuchin blossoms. Serve and enjoy.

Nutrition:

Calories 374

Fat 21g

Protein 44g

Sodium 295mg

Carbohydrate 23.1

Tuna Sandwich

Preparation time: 15 minutes

Cooking time: 0 minutes

Servings: 1

Ingredients:

- 2 slices whole-grain bread

- 1 6-oz. can low sodium tuna in water, in its juice

- 2 tsp Yogurt (1.5% fat) or low-fat mayonnaise

- 1 medium tomato, diced

- ½ small sweet onion, finely diced

- Lettuce leaves

Directions:

1. Toast whole grain bread slices. Mix tuna, yogurt, or mayonnaise, diced tomato, and onion. Cover a toasted bread with lettuce leaves and spread the tuna mixture on the sandwich. Spread tuna mixed on toasted bread with lettuce leaves. Place another disc as a cover on top. Enjoy the sandwich.

Nutrition:

Calories 235

Fat 3g

Protein 27.8g

Sodium 350mg

Carbohydrate 25.9

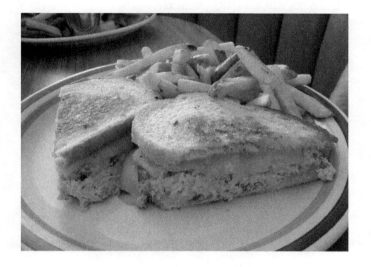

Fruited Quinoa Salad

Preparation time: 15 minutes

Cooking time: 0 minutes

Servings: 2

Ingredients:

- 2 cups cooked quinoa

- 1 mango, sliced and peeled

- 1 cup strawberry, quartered

- ½ cup blueberries

- 2 tablespoon pine nuts

- Chopped mint leave for garnish

- Lemon vinaigrette:

- ¼ cup olive oil

- ¼ cup apple cider vinegar

- Zest of lemon

- 3 tablespoon lemon juice

- 1 teaspoon sugar

Directions:

1. For the Lemon Vinaigrette, whisk olive oil, apple cider vinegar, lemon zest and juice, and sugar to a

bowl; set aside. Combine quinoa, mango strawberries, blueberries, and pine nuts in a large bowl. Stir the lemon vinaigrette and garnish with mint. Serve and enjoy!

Nutrition:
Calories 425
Carbohydrates 76.1g
Proteins 11.3g
Fat 10.9
Sodium 16mg

Turkey Wrap

Preparation time: 15 minutes

Cooking time: 0 minutes

Servings: 2

Ingredients:

- 2 slices of low-fat Turkey breast (deli-style)

- 4 tablespoon non-fat cream cheese

- ½ cup lettuce leaves

- ½ cup carrots, slice into a stick

- 2 Homemade wraps or store-bought whole-wheat tortilla wrap

Directions:

1. Prepare all the ingredients. Spread 2 tablespoons of non-fat cream cheese on each wrap. Arrange lettuce leaves, then add a slice of turkey breast; a slice of carrots stick on top. Roll and cut into half. Serve and enjoy!

Nutrition:

Calories 224

Carbohydrates 35g

Protein 10.3g

Fat 3.8g

Sodium 293mg

Chicken Wrap

Preparation time: 15 minutes

Cooking time: 15 minutes

Servings: 2

Ingredients:

- 1 tablespoon extra- virgin olive oil

- Lemon juice, divided into 3 parts

- 2 cloves garlic, minced

- 1 lb. boneless skinless chicken breasts

- ½ cup non- fat plain Greek yogurt

- ½ teaspoon paprika

- Pinch of salt and pepper

- Hot sauce to taste

- Pita bread

- Tomato slice

Directions:

1. For the marinade, whisk 1 tablespoon olive oil, juice of 2 lemons, garlic, salt, and pepper in a bowl. Add chicken breasts to the marinade and place it into a large Ziploc. Let marinate for 30 mins. to 4 hours.

2. For the yogurt sauce, mix yogurt, hot sauce, and the remaining lemon juice season with paprika and a pinch of salt and pepper.

3. Warm skillet over medium heat and coat it with oil. Add chicken breast and cook until golden brown and cook about 8 minutes per side. Remove from pan and rest for few minutes, then slice.

4. To a piece of pita bread, add lettuce, tomato, and chicken slices. Drizzle with the prepared spicy yogurt sauce. Serve and enjoy!

Nutrition:
Calories 348
Carbohydrates 8.7g
Proteins 56g
Fat 10.2g
Sodium 198mg

Veggie Wrap

Preparation time: 15 minutes

Cooking time: 0 minutes

Servings: 2

Ingredients:

- 2 Homemade wraps or any flour tortillas

- ½ cup spinach

- 1/2 cup alfalfa sprouts

- ½ cup avocado, sliced thinly

- 1 medium tomato, sliced thinly

- ½ cup cucumber, sliced thinly

- Pinch of salt and pepper

Directions:

1. Put 2 tablespoons of cream cheese on each tortilla. Layer each veggie according to your liking. Pinch of salt and pepper. Roll and cut into half. Serve and Enjoy!

Nutrition:

Calories 249

Carbohydrates 12.3g

Protein 5.7g

Fat 21.5g

Sodium 169mg

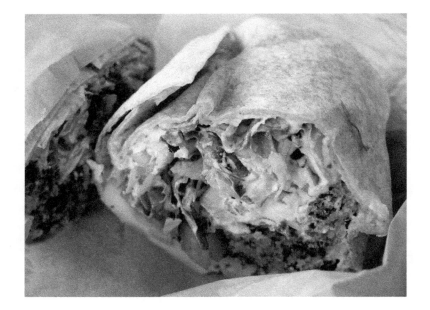

Salmon Wrap

Preparation time: 15 minutes

Cooking time: 0 minutes

Servings: 1

Ingredients:

- 2 oz. Smoke Salmon

- 2 teaspoon low-fat cream cheese

- ½ medium-size red onion, finely sliced

- ½ teaspoon fresh basil or dried basil

- Pinch of pepper

- Arugula leaves

- 1 Homemade wrap or any whole-meal tortilla

Directions:

1. Warm wraps or tortilla into a heated pan or oven. Combine cream cheese, basil, pepper, and spread into the tortilla. Top with salmon, arugula, and sliced onion. Roll up and slice. Serve and Enjoy!

Nutrition:

Calories 151

Carbohydrates 19.2g

Protein 10.4g

Fat 3.4g

Sodium 316mg

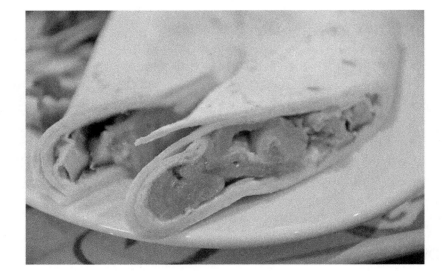

Dill Chicken Salad

Preparation time: 15 minutes
Cooking time: 15 minutes
Servings: 3
Ingredients:

- 1 tablespoon unsalted butter

- 1 small onion, diced

- 2 cloves garlic, minced

- 500g boneless skinless chicken breasts

Salad:

- 2/3 cup Fat-free yogurt

- ¼ cup mayonnaise light

- 2 large shallots, minced

- ½ cup fresh dill, finely chopped

Directions:

1. Dissolve the butter over medium heat in a wide pan. Sauté onion and garlic in the butter and chicken breasts. Put water to cover the chicken breasts by 1 inch. Bring to boil. Cover and reduce the heat to a bare simmer.

2. Cook within 8 to 10 minutes or until the chicken is cooked through. Cool thoroughly. The shred chicken finely using 2 forks. Set aside. Whisk yogurt and mayonnaise. Then toss with the chicken. Add shallots and dill. Mix again all. Serve and Enjoy!

Nutrition:

Calories 253

Carbohydrates 9g

Protein 33.1g

Fat 9.5g

Sodium 236mg

Side Dishes

Turmeric Endives

Preparation time: 10 minutes

Cooking time: 20 minutes

Servings: 4

Ingredients:

- 2 endives, halved lengthwise

- 2 tablespoons olive oil

- 1 teaspoon rosemary, dried

- ½ teaspoon turmeric powder

- A pinch of black pepper

Directions:

1. Mix the endives with the oil and the other ingredients in a baking pan, toss gently, bake at 400 degrees F within 20 minutes. Serve as a side dish.

Nutrition:

Calories 64

Protein 0.2g

Carbohydrates 0.8g

Fat 7.1g

Fiber 0.6g

Sodium 3mg

Potassium 50mg

Parmesan Endives

Preparation time: 10 minutes

Cooking time: 20 minutes

Servings: 4

Ingredients:

- 4 endives, halved lengthwise

- 1 tablespoon lemon juice

- 1 tablespoon lemon zest, grated

- 2 tablespoons fat-free parmesan, grated

- 2 tablespoons olive oil

- A pinch of black pepper

Directions:

1. In a baking dish, combine the endives with the lemon juice and the other ingredients except for the parmesan and toss. Sprinkle the parmesan on top, bake the endives at 400 degrees F for 20 minutes, and serve.

Nutrition:

Calories 71

Protein 0.9g

Carbohydrates 2.2g

Fat 7.1g

Fiber 0.9g

Sodium 71mg

Potassium 88mg

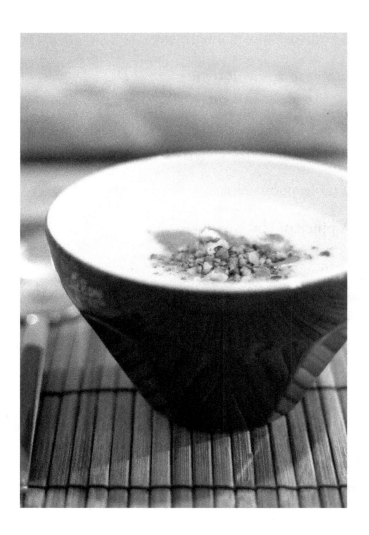

Lemon Asparagus

Preparation time: 10 minutes

Cooking time: 20 minutes

Servings: 4

Ingredients:

- 1-pound asparagus, trimmed

- 2 tablespoons basil pesto

- 1 tablespoon lemon juice

- A pinch of black pepper

- 3 tablespoons olive oil

- 2 tablespoons cilantro, chopped

Directions:

1. Arrange the asparagus n a lined baking sheet, add the pesto and the other ingredients, toss, bake at 400 degrees F within 20 minutes. Serve as a side dish.

Nutrition:

Calories 114

Protein 2.6g

Carbohydrates 4.5g

Fat 10.7g

Fiber 2.4g

Sodium 3mg

Potassium 240mg

Lime Carrots

Preparation time: 10 minutes

Cooking time: 30 minutes

Servings: 4

Ingredients:

- 1-pound baby carrots, trimmed

- 1 tablespoon sweet paprika

- 1 teaspoon lime juice

- 3 tablespoons olive oil

- A pinch of black pepper

- 1 teaspoon sesame seeds

Directions:

1. Arrange the carrots on a lined baking sheet, add the paprika and the other ingredients except for the sesame seeds, toss, bake at 400 degrees F within 30 minutes. Divide the carrots between plates, sprinkle sesame seeds on top and serve as a side dish.

Nutrition:

Calories 139

Protein 1.1g

Carbohydrates 10.5g

Fat 11.2g

4g fiber

Sodium 89mg

Potassium 313mg

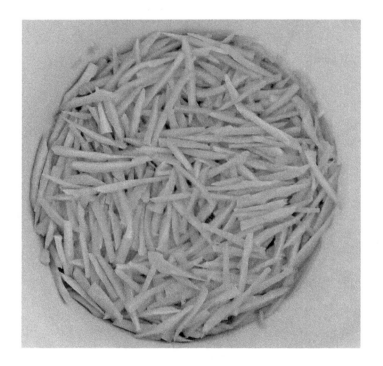

Garlic Potato Pan

Preparation time: 10 minutes

Cooking time: 1 hour

Servings: 8

Ingredients:

- 1-pound gold potatoes, peeled and cut into wedges

- 2 tablespoons olive oil

- 1 red onion, chopped

- 2 garlic cloves, minced

- 2 cups coconut cream

- 1 tablespoon thyme, chopped

- ¼ teaspoon nutmeg, ground

- ½ cup low-fat parmesan, grated

Directions:

1. Warm-up a pan with the oil over medium heat, put the onion plus the garlic, and sauté for 5 minutes. Add the potatoes and brown them for 5 minutes more.

2. Add the cream and the rest of the ingredients, toss gently, bring to a simmer and cook over medium

heat within 40 minutes more. Divide the mix between plates and serve as a side dish.

Nutrition:

Calories 230

Protein 3.6g

Carbohydrates 14.3g

Fat 19.1g

Fiber 3.3g

Cholesterol 6mg

Sodium 105mg

Potassium 426mg

Balsamic Cabbage

Preparation time: 10 minutes

Cooking time: 20 minutes

Servings: 4

Ingredients:

- 1-pound green cabbage, roughly shredded

- 2 tablespoons olive oil

- A pinch of black pepper

- 1 shallot, chopped

- 2 garlic cloves, minced

- 2 tablespoons balsamic vinegar

- 2 teaspoons hot paprika

- 1 teaspoon sesame seeds

Directions:

1. Heat-up a pan with the oil over medium heat, add the shallot and the garlic, and sauté for 5 minutes. Add the cabbage and the other ingredients, toss, cook over medium heat for 15 minutes, divide between plates and serve.

Nutrition:

Calories 100

Protein 1.8g

Carbohydrates 8.2g

Fat 7.5g

Fiber 3g

Sodium 22mg

Potassium 225mg

Chili Broccoli

Preparation time: 10 minutes

Cooking time: 30 minutes

Servings: 4

Ingredients:

- 2 tablespoons olive oil

- 1-pound broccoli florets

- 2 garlic cloves, minced

- 2 tablespoons chili sauce

- 1 tablespoon lemon juice

- A pinch of black pepper

- 2 tablespoons cilantro, chopped

Directions:

1. In a baking pan, combine the broccoli with the oil, garlic, and the other, toss a bit, and bake at 400 degrees F for 30 minutes. Divide the mix between plates and serve as a side dish.

Nutrition:

Calories 103

Protein 3.4g

Carbohydrates 8.3gz

7.4g fat

3g fiber

Sodium 229mg

Potassium 383mg

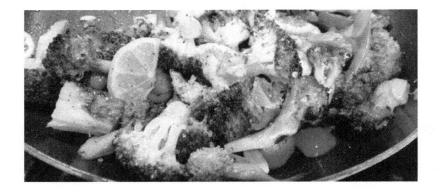

Hot Brussels Sprouts

Preparation time: 10 minutes

Cooking time: 25 minutes

Servings: 4

Ingredients:

- 1 tablespoon olive oil

- 1-pound Brussels sprouts, trimmed and halved

- 2 garlic cloves, minced

- ½ cup low-fat mozzarella, shredded

- A pinch of pepper flakes, crushed

Directions:

1. In a baking dish, combine the sprouts with the oil and the other ingredients except for the cheese and toss. Sprinkle the cheese on top, introduce in the oven and bake at 400 degrees F for 25 minutes. Divide between plates and serve as a side dish.

Nutrition:

Calories 111

Protein 10g

Carbohydrates 11.6g

Fat 3.9g

Fiber 5g

Cholesterol 4mg

Sodium 209mg

Potassium 447mg

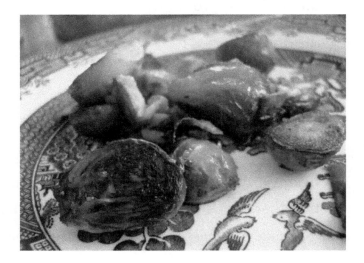

Paprika Brussels Sprouts

Preparation time: 10 minutes

Cooking time: 25 minutes

Servings: 4

Ingredients:

- 2 tablespoons olive oil

- 1-pound Brussels sprouts, trimmed and halved

- 3 green onions, chopped

- 2 garlic cloves, minced

- 1 tablespoon balsamic vinegar

- 1 tablespoon sweet paprika

- A pinch of black pepper

Directions:

1. In a baking pan, combine the Brussels sprouts with the oil and the other ingredients, toss and bake at 400 degrees F within 25 minutes. Divide the mix between plates and serve.

Nutrition:

Calories 121

Protein 4.4g

Carbohydrates 12.6g

Fat 7.6g

Fiber 5.2g

Sodium 31mg

Potassium 521mg

Creamy Cauliflower Mash

Preparation time: 10 minutes

Cooking time: 25 minutes

Servings: 4

Ingredients:

- 2 pounds cauliflower florets

- ½ cup of coconut milk

- A pinch of black pepper

- ½ cup low-fat sour cream

- 1 tablespoon cilantro, chopped

- 1 tablespoon chives, chopped

Directions:

1. Put the cauliflower in a pot, add water to cover, bring to a boil over medium heat, cook for 25 minutes and drain. Mash the cauliflower, add the milk, black pepper, and the cream, whisk well, divide between plates, sprinkle the rest of the ingredients on top, and serve.

Nutrition:

Calories 188

Protein 6.1g

Carbohydrates 15g

Fat 13.4g

Fiber 6.4g

Cholesterol 13mg

Sodium 88mg

Potassium 811mg

Avocado, Tomato, and Olives Salad

Preparation time: 5 minutes

Cooking time: 0 minutes

Servings: 4

Ingredients:

- 2 tablespoons olive oil

- 2 avocados, cut into wedges

- 1 cup kalamata olives, pitted and halved

- 1 cup tomatoes, cubed

- 1 tablespoon ginger, grated

- A pinch of black pepper

- 2 cups baby arugula

- 1 tablespoon balsamic vinegar

Directions:

1. In a bowl, combine the avocados with the kalamata and the other ingredients, toss and serve as a side dish.

Nutrition:

Calories 320

Protein 3g

Carbohydrates 13.9g

Fat 30.4g

Fiber 8.7g

Sodium 305mg

Potassium 655mg

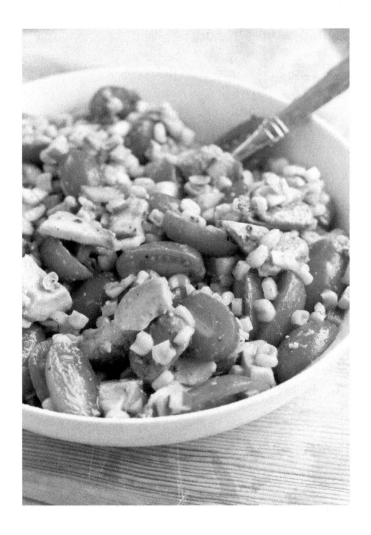